CDA DENTISTRY INTERVIEW PREPARATION

CDA Dentistry Interview Preparation

James Walker

Maximello Publishers
868, 141-6200 McKay Ave.
Burnaby, BC V5H 4M9
http://www.maximello.com

James Walker
Visit my website at http://www.cdainterviews.com

Printed in Canada

Cover design by David Wang

Walker, James, 1984-
CDA dentistry interview preparation / James Walker.

ISBN 978-0-9813492-2-0

1. Dental schools--Canada--Entrance examinations--Study guides. 2. Interviewing. I. Title.

RK57.W25 2009 617.60076 C2009-905597-X

Table of Contents

Chapter 1 Introduction

The Canadian Dental Association interview for admission into a Canadian dental school is critical for candidates for the dentistry program. The stakes are high in these dentistry interviews as the future, career, and years invested in academic and extracurricular preparation are at stake. The competition is stiff between many highly qualified applicants. The interview is often the determining factor among the many competitive applications of high GPA and DAT scores. The candidates also have a limited number of two attempts at the interview in his or her whole life time at a particular school. A thorough preparation for the dentistry interview is crucial and this book will provide information to prepare you for your interview, show you an approach to answer CDA interview questions, guide you in your preparation and leave you feeling confident and prepared for your interview.

Chapter 2 CDA Interview

The Canadian Dental Association interview for admission into a Canadian dental school is a standardized interview. The questions are created by the CDA and sent to the all the schools so that even the schools receive the interview questions within a few days of the actual interview. All the schools have the same set of interview questions across the country and the interviewers select questions from the interview question set. Hence, a dentistry applicant can use the score from one dental school for another dental school application. The interview is structured the same every year and is suppose to last about 30 to 45 minutes. There will always be about seven questions and the questions are aimed at testing one or more of the competencies that have been outlined by CDA as qualities that they desire in a dentist. These qualities are publically stated and are qualities generally expected of a health care professional. The interviewer is actively looking and evaluating these qualities in every question. The interviewee should aim to demonstrate that they possess these qualities when answering the questions. The applicant should recognize certain qualities the question is targeting, state the qualities they possess and support the statement with past experiences. In general, the questions are designed to target mainly one competency each and it is usually fairly obvious to an interviewee who is aware and looking for the competencies being tested. The applicant should have past experiences that demonstrate each of the competencies prepared before the interview because it is very difficult to think of examples spontaneously during the interview, especially under the stress of the interview and the need to deliver the experience in an organized and clear manner. The best way to prepare for the CDA interview is to start preparing early so you allow yourself time to brainstorm and recall past experiences that demonstrate the qualities desired by CDA. You should use a chart that shows each of the qualities and complete the chart so that you have at least three experiences you can relay to the interviewer when the opportunity to demonstrate the competency arises. Once you've brainstormed the past experiences, you will need to practice organizing and delivering the past experience as a coherent, clear, and organized story. You may want to write out the story of your past experiences and practice delivering the story in front of a video camera. Then evaluate the videotape of yourself searching for strength and weaknesses and work on the areas that you can improve. A useful structure for organizing your past experiences is known as the SAR structure. This structure is recommended for any situational type of question where you need to relay a past experience to support your answer. The acronyms SAR represent Situation, Action, and Result. You begin by setting the stage of the story and briefly explain the situation you were faced with and this will lead to your analysis of the situation and what you did in the situation. Finally, you end the story with a strong conclusion by stating the results of your action and demonstrate that your actions resolved the problem outlined at the beginning of the story or the lessons you've gleaned from the story. It is important to have stories in which you've failed and learned something because it is common to encounter questions in which they will search and directly ask for situations in which you've failed at something and want to know what you've gained or learned from the situation.

The Importance of the Interview

The interview is very important for entry into dentistry. All the applicants who are invited to an interview are selected and have submitted highly competitive applications. The main determining factor for admission into dentistry becomes the interview. Applicants can no longer rely on a strong GPA or DAT scores anymore and the interview can be "make or break" for entering dentistry. The interviews introduce a "human" component to the often impersonal application process. The interview is the first time the dental school can see and talk to the applicant in person and to evaluate the applicant as more than just a paper application. The softer skills and people skills are vital in health care professions such as dentistry. The interview is an opportunity for the dental schools to evaluate social and soft skills of the applicant and is a critical component for dental school admission.

CDA Interview Format

The CDA interview is a structured and standardized interview in which all the questions have been created by the CDA and sent to all the dental schools. The CDA interview is approximately 35 minutes in length. The applicant is interviewed by a panel of two to three interviewers that have undergone a CDA interview training workshop. The interviewers are general practitioners, faculty members, or dental students. It is important to note that the interviewers do not have access to the candidate's file. Hence, the score the interviewers assign to the applicant is solely based on the answers in response to the questions. The interviewers will ask seven questions. There are two versions of each question. The interviewers pick from a list of questions provided by the CDA. The dental schools receive the questions within a few days of the actual interview. Since all the questions and administration are standardized by the CDA, a CDA interview is equivalent for any dental school in Canada. An applicant is allowed to use a score from one dental school for another dental school so the applicant doesn't need to travel to another dental school for an interview. The catch is that you don't know the score of the interview that you transfer to another dental school. The applicant is also limited to only two CDA interviews per school.

Types of Questions for the CDA Interview

There are two types of questions in CDA interviews. The types of questions are either situational questions or patterned behavior descriptions.

Situational questions ask the candidate what they would do in a hypothetical situation.

Patterned behavior descriptions are the type of question in which the interviewer asks about a past behavior. The assumption for this type of question is that past experiences and behavior are good predictors of future behavior.

One of the objectives of the CDA interview is to select applicants that are suitable as dentists. The CDA has constructed a list of qualities they believe are important for a dentist. As a result, the CDA evaluates the applicant on these qualities in the interview. There are seven qualities or "competencies" as referred to by the CDA and as a result there are seven questions, each question testing one of the seven competencies. Competencies are behaviors characterized by performance in realistic circumstances appropriate to your life experience. In other words, the CDA interview is assessing whether the applicant possesses personal characteristics that will enable the person to behave appropriately as a health professional.

The seven competencies are sensitivity to others, self control, tact and diplomacy, integrity, judgment and analysis, conscientiousness, and communication.

Sensitivity to others is being aware of and responsive to the feelings of others. As a dentist is health care professional dealing with patients who are vulnerable, they need to exercise compassion and empathy to best help the patient. Patients commonly visit their dentist with apprehensions, fear, nervousness, and anxiety and being empathic with the patients is important to putting the patient at ease and providing quality dental health care.

Self control is being in control or having restraint of oneself or one's actions, feelings, and thoughts. This competency is part of being a professional that provides specialized services based on the trust and confidence provided by the patient. A professional cannot be reckless and must possess a certain level of self discipline to provide quality care and ensure the safety of the patient.

Tact and diplomacy go hand in hand. Tact is having a keen sense of what to say or do to avoid giving offence and is possessing skill in dealing with difficult or delicate situations. Diplomacy is the skill in managing negotiations, handling people and etc. so that there is little or no ill will. These skills are important in maintaining positive clinician and patient relationship.

Integrity is the adherence to moral and ethical principles, having a soundness of moral character and being honest. The fiduciary relationship between a patient and the dentist demands a level of integrity for the entrusting his or her health to the clinician.

Judgment and analysis follow one another where analysis is the process of studying the nature of something or of determining its essential features and their relations. Judgment is the ability to make a decision or form an opinion objectively, authoritatively, and wisely; especially in matters affecting action. A certain level of intelligence and analytical skill is required for the duties and responsibilities of a health care professional.

Conscientiousness is characterized by showing care, attention, and effort. A significant amount of work performed by a dentist requires a high level of attention and care. A certain level of conscientiousness is required to learn and to perform the tasks required of a dentist.

Communication is defined didactically as the imparting or interchange of thoughts, opinions, or information by speech, writing, or signs. This definition serves to remind the applicant that despite the interview being a verbal form of communication, the interviewers are also searching for other mediums of communication including written reports, presentations, and ideas outside of science and dentistry.

Chapter 3 Preparation for the Interview

The most important thing that you can do to help your interview performance is to prepare. The types of questions asked in a CDA interview will be very difficult to answer on the spot. It is difficult to recall good examples one after another for several consecutive questions probing different competencies. You should be able to tie in real life examples for both the situational and pattern behavior type of questions. Hence, it is important to prepare for this type of interview by brainstorming past experiences related to the seven competencies. Once you have brainstormed past experiences for each of the seven competencies, you will have content that you can use to answer any of the seven questions they ask you. Sometimes, brainstorming can be difficult, especially when you are analyzing yourself. So you should enlist family and friends to help brainstorm because they may notice or recall things you have long forgotten or shrugged off as unimportant but perfectly illustrate the competencies.

The brainstorming of past experiences to match the seven competencies should begin about three months before the actual interview. This will allow you time to brainstorm new past experiences, sculpt and practice your responses, and give you time to improve and practice with mock interviews.

To help you with your brainstorming, the next few pages have been designed to organize your brainstorming. There is ample room to write your past experiences. When brainstorming for past experiences for each competency, write any ideas that come to your mind and strive to fill the whole page. Spend at least five minutes writing nonstop filling in past experiences for each competency.

CDA Interview Preparation: Situation Brainstorming

Competency: Sensitivity to Others

Definition: Aware of and responsive to the feelings of others

Situation Examples:

Competency: Self Control

Definition: Control or restraint of oneself or one's actions, feelings, etc.

Situation Examples:

Competency:	Tact and Diplomacy	
Definition:	Tact:	A keen sense of what to say or do to avoid giving offence; skill in dealing with difficult or delicate situations.
	Diplomacy:	Skill in managing negotiations, handling people, etc., so that there is little or no ill will

Situation Examples:

Competency: Integrity

Definition: Adherence to moral and ethical principles; soundness of moral character; honesty

Situation Examples:

Competency: Judgment and Analysis

Definition:

Judgment: The ability to make a decision or form an opinion objectively, authoritatively, and wisely, especially in matters affecting action.

Analysis: The process of studying the nature of something or of determining its essential features and their relations

Situation Examples:

Competency: Conscientiousness

Definition: Characterized by showing care, attention, effort

Situation Examples:

Competency: Communication

Definition: The imparting or interchange of thoughts, opinions, or information by speech, writing, or signs

Situation Examples:

After you have finished brainstorming ideas, you will select three of the past experiences that you feel best illustrates the competency. The next step is to carve a well organized, concise, and compelling response with each of these past experiences. You need to create a story and paint a picture with your past experiences to illustrate the competencies. A useful organizational structure to construct your answers and still have the natural storytelling like effect and is easy to remember and most importantly recall during the interview is the SAR structure. The SAR structure stands for Situation, Action and Response. You begin your response by describing the situation you were dealing with and the dilemma or problem you were faced with. Then move onto to describe the action or the factors that you considered and the specific actions you took to resolve the problem or situation. Remember to focus on tasks that you performed and not to dilute your answer with actions done by other people. The interviewer is interested in you and your actions. After describing what you did to resolve the issue, this naturally leads to the result of your actions. The outcome of your actions could be positive and you can triumphantly describe the benefits of your action or if the outcome was negative you can describe the lessons you've learned and how it has made you more aware of yourself and efforts you've done to improve yourself. Not everyone is perfect and having some past experiences that illustrate past failures and what you've learned from them will often become necessary in answering some of the interview questions. Some of the most difficult interview questions will ask for your weaknesses or worst experiences. Everyone has areas of improvement so you can't be honest and still escape these questions with blanket statements of perfectionisms. In preparing responses for weaknesses be sure to have clear lessons and efforts to overcome these challenges. But with some planning these traditionally difficult questions will become just another question that you have prepared to answer.

The next step in preparing for the interview is to practice interviewing by doing mock interviews. You can inquire with the career services department in your university or pre-dental interview help around campus for mock interview practice. You can also enlist a panel of family and friends and have them ask you interview questions. There are many interviews in this book that you can use to practice interviewing with different people. An equivalent to nine CDA interviews worth of practice and mock interviews are available near the end of the book. After you have practiced your mock interview, make sure you get feedback. Feedback is the most important method to find areas for improvement and to raise your interview performance. Have you friends and family comment on your performance or videotape yourself. Videotaping your interviews is very effective because you can review your interview many times and you'll often spot areas of improvement each time. Also, you are often your hardest critic and to enlist yourself by using a video camera is an invaluable tool. A tip with the video camera is to fast forward your tape and any mannerisms that you are normally oblivious will become exaggerated and very obvious. You might notice mannerisms such as distracting gestures, fidgeting, awkward body language, and using filler words such "um," "like," or "ah."

Part of the interview preparation is planning out your outfit that you'll wear on interview day. As much as clothing is associated with fashion, the dentistry interview is not the time to make a fashion statement. Your physical appearance is the first impression that you will make. The health profession is still a conservative profession so you want to dress accordingly. In general, a dark suit is recommended for men. Women have more options in terms of clothing and should still be conservative. In general skirts should not be above the knees, dress shoes should be closed toed and scented products used sparingly. Accessories should be modest so men should not elect distracting ties, or tie clips. Proper hygiene is expected so men should groom their facial hair. Overall, the outfit should be aimed to look professional and avoid anything that would be distracting. One last note about the outfit is to practice wearing the outfit before the interview to avoid wardrobe malfunctions.

Chapter 4 The Interview Day

What Happens on Interview Day?

CDA interviews involve the applicant answering a set of standardized questions. The interviewee will generally sign in and convene in a waiting room where they will be called to an interview room. The interview rooms are usually small and cozy. There will be two or three interviewers composed of dentists, dental students, and faculty. The interviews generally last for about half an hour to an hour. At the end of the interview, the applicants are released either to go home or activities such as tours or presentations arranged by the school of dentistry.

What to Do During the Interview?

The first thing you should the moment you enter the interview room is make eye contact and acknowledge the interviewer by name and introduce yourself. Then shake hands with interviewers with a firm but not bone crushing handshake. Be sure to maintain eye contact and smile at appropriate times. Smiling is the easiest and most effective thing you can do to develop rapport with the interviewer. Unfortunately, many times the interviewee is too nervous and often forget to smile and even worse by frowning or be stern faced during the interview. You want to look and feel natural and avoid looking stiff or tense. In addition, you want to maintain proper posture by not slouching. You also want to be mindful of negative body language such as crossing your arms, fidgeting, touching things on the table, and crossing your legs. When you speak you want to project clarity in your voice and pay attention to maintain moderate speed and volume. Anxiety often makes people unconsciously speed up. The interview room is usually small so the volume of voice is generally not too loud otherwise a loud voice can overwhelm the room and be uncomfortable for the interviewers.

When presenting your responses you want to be genuine and provide sincere answers. Acting or providing artificial answers are very obvious and may be detrimental to your score and hamper rapport development with the interviewer. So you shouldn't try to memorize answers for the fear of forgetting and to avoid providing stilted and unnatural answers. Injecting humor in your interview can help loosen the atmosphere and build rapport. However, only use humor if it comes naturally and if can remain professional. A useful tip is to pause and take a deep breath when needed to help you relax and not tense up.

After hearing the question, don't rush to answer the question even if you know what to say. You want to give a measured and deliberate pause before you answer to give you time to mentally prepare and to avoid appearing rushed. Take the few moments immediately after hearing the question to think over the question. In your mind, try to isolate the competency that the question reflects and use it as a guide for your answer. Before launching into an answer, always have a basic idea of what you want to say, otherwise you get bogged down and risk being circular in your response. A useful structure to organize your response is to structure your answer like an oral essay with a clear answer, supporting arguments, and conclusion. Your answer should aim to be clear, complete, thoughtful, logical, and sincere.

There may be a time when you don't know the answer to the question. Be rest assured that you are allowed time to think before answering. You can tell the interviewer that you need a moment to think of the answer. It is better to have a minute silence than a minute of "umm..." so do not be worried that you are enveloped with silence while you think of a response. Be aware of the temptation to make up something up, especially for pattern behavior questions. If necessary, you can say what you would do if you cannot think of a past experience. If you continue to struggle with a particular question, you have a choice of moving to the next question and returning to the question later. This alternative will give you time to think of a response while you answer other questions and maybe find inspiration for the question while you're answering another question.

When you're answering the questions, the interviewers will try to guide you if they feel you are getting lost. Remember that for all of the questions, the why is more important than the what. You should always be honest because there are no right answers. You should always justify your response despite your belief. The interviewers are especially interested in your thought process and logic. In order to substantiate your response and make it more concrete, you want to incorporate a real life example whenever appropriate.

What to Do After the Interview?

After the interview, shake hands, say thank you, and good bye, and leave the interview room. Do not dawdle after the interview but leave courteously. When you're done it is inevitable to self-analyze your performance and to reflect on the length of time of the interview. Some may worry that spending too little time was being too brief or spending too much time was being verbose. As you speak with other applicants you may become even more worried and confused as you get a mixture of stories. You shouldn't think too much about your performance as the only valid indicator of your performance is the feedback from the dental school and the admission result. Feel rest assured that most dental students don't know how well did they did on their interview and the length of the interview may range from 25 minutes to 45 minutes but the length of the interview is unrelated to the performance.

If you have any concerns about discriminatory behavior, inappropriate questions, or poor interview techniques, report to the admissions office before leaving. Remember, you are only graded on your answers to the seven CDA questions.

Chapter 5 CDA Interview Experiences: Stories from Applicants

Interview at the University of British Columbia

I had my interview in mid morning at 11 AM and walked up to the new, gleaming Oral Health Centre made from glass and metal and resplendent with the latest architectural designs. I opened the glass door framed with metal and immediately encountered a smiling woman behind a small wooden desk ready to check me in for the interview. I gave her my name and verified against my driver's license and was instructed to go upstairs. Immediately behind the friendly lady was spiraling staircase. As I was walking up the stairs I saw an applicant who just finished her interview and she left smiling and wished me well. I entered the second floor to witness a modernly furnished floor with hardwood floor. Immediately above me was a multicolored chandelier and in front of me was large wooden reception desk. To the left of me was a lounge and eating area arranged comfortably and reminiscent of Starbucks type of layout. A lady met me at the second floor and escorted me to the right side where I noticed a smaller area with two rows of about eight leather armchairs on either side facing each other. I came in early and there was one person sitting near the middle of the row facing me. I walked and sat on the closer row and faced her. We chatted and shared our mutual feelings of nervousness as well waited for the interview. Another jaunty fellow came out of his interview smiling and reassured us that the interviewers are nice and we shouldn't worry. We waited on the armchairs and slowly the rest of the interviewees came and we chatted, encouraged each other, and shared being nervous together despite the reassurance given by the people who just finished their interviews. The interviewees came in and took seats near the middle of the row and expanded to fill both rows. As we waited a lady walks out from a hallway behind the reception desk and calls out a name and one of the applicants leave with the lady and they both walked into the hallway and disappeared around a corner. The rest of the applicants cheered at the applicant who was called. Now the attention of the group of applicants was to look at the hallway in anticipation of the next applicant to be called upon. A few of the applicants needed to use the washroom, me included. After a few more minutes, another applicant was called in the same fashion and disappeared around the bend of the hallway with the remaining applicants cheering for him. The sporadically spaced times to wait punctuated by interviewers appearing and taking the applicant away continued and the cheering existed but became weaker due to the smaller group of people that remained. I waited and couldn't help but notice that almost all the applicants have been called in except for me a couple of other applicants. The anxiety mounts as the waiting continues near the end. We hear a pair of clacking sounds that suggests a pair of high heels coming from around the corner of the hallway. The clacking of the high heels becomes progressively louder until a bright, smiling young lady appears out of the hallway. She called my name and I leaped to my feet to simultaneously realize that being called has brought me relief in ending the anxiety building wait and sudden apprehension of the imminent beginning of the interview. I followed her down the hallway I saw so many applicants disappeared before and to my surprise I was lead down a labyrinth of hallways that turned and crossed. I was thoroughly lost but simply followed the interviewer as she began some small talk. Finally, she stops in front of a door in the middle of a long hallway of doors. I didn't know what to expect when she opened the door. She let me into a small room and another interviewer was sitting behind a small desk. The interviewer got up to introduce himself and escorted me to a chair on the other side of the desk. The lady interviewer sat on the side of the desk while the male interviewer sat directly across from me. I noticed the age difference between the two interviewers; the lady was not much older than me while the male interviewer was in his 50's. I mentally guessed that the older interviewer was an established dentist while the younger interviewer was probably dental student. Shortly after the greetings they introduced themselves and confirmed my guess. The younger interviewer was about a year from finishing her dental program and the older interviewer was a dentist who also did some clinical teaching at the university. We talked and joked for a few more minutes before the interviewers pulled out their clipboards, explained the procedure of the CDA interview and began asking the CDA interview questions. The younger interviewer started asking an interview question by reading off the clipboard and jotted notes while I answered. Then the older interviewer would repeat the same routine and the two interviewers alternated in asking questions. The cycle of alternative repeated about four times and all the CDA interview questions were answered. The interview ended with some more conversation and the younger interviewer again escorted me back to the waiting area. The UBC Dentistry interview also contained a second component in the afternoon. I had lunch with a few of the other applicants and waited for the second part of the interview scheduled after lunch. The applicants convened in a lecture hall and an instructor gave us a thirty minute briefing of Problem Based Learning and we were suppose to participated in a PBL as the second part of the interview. We were divided into groups and went to an assigned room. The room was a small classroom with half a dozen tables and a blackboard. A small round of self introductions followed by the PBL instructor handing out a problem and we were let free to tackle the problem as a group while the PBL instructor sat in the back to observe, take notes, and evaluate. The group tackled the problem for thirty minutes or so before the PBL instructor provided more information on the case and this was repeated a couple of times before the PBL instructor dismissed the group and officially ended the long day of interview at UBC.

Interview at the University of Alberta

It was beautiful sunny morning as I walked through the crisp morning air to the dentistry building at the University of Alberta. I walked into a stone historical building and followed the signs that lead me down a hallway to a small lecture hall with cushioned seats where I signed in at the front of the lecture room. I took a seat at a third filled room and looked around. The seats were filled by men in black suits and women in business formal wear waiting for something. I sat and noticed that people were being called away by current dental students. After sitting and waiting for a while I was called by a young male dentistry student. I escorted me to the third floor of the building and took me to two large wooden doors that were slightly opened. My escort told me that the door in front of us was my interview room and waited for me to go in. All I saw was a gleam of light coming out of an ominously large pair of wooden doors that could easily have been an entrance to a large lecture hall. The thought of interviewing in a lecture hall was daunting and I hesitated to enter the room but the escort was waiting and encouraged me to enter the room. I entered to room not knowing what to expect and I was surprised by the bright light of the room. The next thing that struck me was the small size of the room. The room was a small waiting area for a dental clinical room with a coffee table in the middle that was completely covered with neatly placed magazines and cushioned chairs around the coffee table. As I made a quick look around the room and I was struck at the close proximity of the three interviewers. A man in his fifties extended his hand to greet me followed by a young girl and a middle age woman. Through the introductions I learned that the man was a practicing dentist, the young girl was a dentistry student, and the middle age woman was an instructor at the dentistry school. The man explained the interview structure will be round robin. I sat down and I was facing the dental student with the man to the left and the middle age woman to the right. The middle age woman began the interview and read the question off her clipboard, followed by the dentistry student and then by the man. This was repeated a couple of times. The man offered an opportunity to add information at the end of the interview. The interview concluded with an exchange of handshakes and I was escorted out of the room where I saw my escort waiting in the hallway. The escort brought me down to the lecture hall where I waited with other interviewees. I noticed some interviewees coming into the room were anxiously waiting for their interview. After a brief period of waiting we were offered a tour of the school of dentistry lead by a dentistry and dental hygiene student. After the tour, the tour guides answered some questions, provided some information on the release of the admissions results and we were summarily dismissed just in time for lunch.

Conclusion

The CDA interview is unique from typical job interviews and the preparations you've completed will equip you with valuable information and prime you to provide insightful and organized responses for your interview. You will be ready for one of the most important interviews in your life. After completing the thorough preparation in this book you can relax, be natural and complete your interview with ease and confidence. I wish best of luck in your interview, admission, career and life.

Practice CDA Style Interview Questions

Flip the page to begin.

Interview #1

1. You are working in a clothing store as a customer service representative. Your supervisor arrives to work drunk. What would you do?

2. Your younger brother has a physics exam next week. He asks you to help him while you are on your way to watch a movie with your friends. What would you do?

3. Tell me a time when you had to convince someone to accomplish a task.

4. When was a time you had to tell the truth even though it was difficult?

5. You are working in a group project for school. One of the group members is always late and doesn't seem to be engaged during group meetings. What would you do?

6. Describe a time when you were faced with a dilemma. How did you handle it? How did things turn out?

7. Your best friend gives you a gift. He later confides in you that he stole the gift. How would you react?

Interview #2

1. Tell us a time when your first method of explaining an idea or instruction did not work and you need to find an alternative method to get the message across.

2. Tell us a time when you had to tell bad news to someone.

3. Given what you know now, what is one thing that you would do differently in your life?

4. You are working at a coffee shop and your supervisor tells you to make the coffee in a way that is slower. What would you do?

5. You are giving a presentation and there is a heckler in the audience. He is constantly stopping you and diverting you from the main part of the presentation. How would you deal with the situation?

6. During university there are times when you had a very heavy course load. Tell me how you handled a very heavy course load.

7. Tell us a time when you made a decision that was unpopular but was the right one.

Interview #3

1. Describe a situation where you felt angry and how you responded.

2. You are going on a fishing trip with a group of friends. You also invite your neighbor who is an international student. When you go pick her up, she is dressed in high heels, a dress and clothing not suitable for fishing. How do you approach the situation?

3. Tell us a time when you proposed an idea that was not well received by a person of higher authority and how you responded.

4. How did you prepare for this interview?

5. You are working at a fast food restaurant and your colleague is cooking hamburger patties on the grill. It is during lunch hour and the team is falling behind on the orders and you noticed that your colleague is rushing such that some of the patties don't seem to be completely cooked. What would you do?

6. Imagine you are shopping at a small grocery store and you saw a middle age lady stick a chocolate bar into her purse. What would you do?

7. Describe a time when you had a lot of work and many personal problems. What did you do to resolve the situation you faced? What would you do differently?

Interview #4

1. If you were planning a trip to climb Mount Everest, how would you prepare for the trip?

2. If you've already attempted to apply for Dentistry twice and didn't get in, what would you do?

3. Tell me a time when you needed to explain a technical or complicated topic in a way that was easy for the other person to understand.

4. Describe a time when you needed to make a decision under pressure and within a short period of time.

5. You are working on a team project and you are asking one of your team members for information that you need to complete your task. However, that team member does not respond to your e-mails. What would you do?

6. You are a manager working at a fast food restaurant and you noticed that one of the employees on your team is working slow and impeding the flow. What would you do?

7. You are working on a class project and you noticed one of the team members is constantly complaining. What would you do?

Interview #5

1. Tell me a time when you needed to organize an event.

2. Describe a time when you need to persuade someone to support you.

3. Tell me about a time when you needed to provide advice to someone.

4. You see a foreign person carrying a suitcase and he appears to be lost. His command of the English language is minimal. What would you do?

5. Tell me about a time when you were treated unfairly by an authority.

6. Your best friend broke up with their boyfriend and is feeling very sad. How do you respond?

7. Describe a time when things did not happen as planned and what you would do differently.

www.ingramcontent.com/pod-product-compliance
Lightning Source LLC
LaVergne TN
LVHW022323200926
848481LV00004B/1403